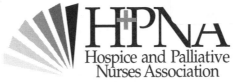

HPNA
Hospice and Palliative
Nurses Association

Compendium of Treatment of End Stage Non-Cancer Diagnoses

Pulmonary

Margaret L. Campbell, RN, PhD, FAAN
Detroit, MI

Patrick Coyne, MSN, APRN, BC-PCM, FAAN
Compendium Editor

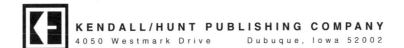

KENDALL/HUNT PUBLISHING COMPANY
4050 Westmark Drive   Dubuque, Iowa 52002

Contents

Expert Reviewers   iv

Disclaimer   v

Introduction   vii

Overview   1

Definitions   2

Pathophysiology   2

Assessment   4

Early Treatment Interventions   7

Later Treatment Interventions   8

Psychosocial   14

Economics   15

Ethics   15

Research Questions   15

Summary   16

Cited References   17

Expert Reviewers

Deena E. Bugge, RNC, CHPN®
Registered Clinical Nurse IV
Virginia Commonwealth University
  Health System
Richmond, VA

Lea Ann Hansen, PharmD, BCOP
Associate Professor of Pharmacy
Virginia Commonwealth University
Richmond, VA

Tamara Sacks, MD
Palliative Medicine Fellow
Virginia Commonwealth University
Richmond, VA

Patrick J. Coyne, MSN, APRN, BC-PCM, FAAN
Clinical Nurse Specialist for
  Pain/Palliative Care
Clinical Director of Thomas Palliative
  Care Program
Virginia Commonwealth
  University/Massey Cancer Center
Richmond, VA

Judy Lentz, RN, MSN, NHA
Chief Executive Officer
Hospice and Palliative Nurses Association
Pittsburgh, PA

Dena Jean Sutermaster, RN, MSN, CHPN®
Director of Education/Research
Hospice and Palliative Nurses Association
Pittsburgh, PA

Disclaimer

HPNA will not be held liable or responsible for individual treatments, specific plans of care or patient and family outcomes. This compendium is intended for professional educational purposes only.

Introduction

As palliative care nursing continues to expand within the illness continuum and clearly beyond the population of oncology, nurses delivering this care must be knowledgeable in the current research and appropriate treatment strategies. This series of modules is designed to serve as a resource in constructing an appropriate plan of care for individuals and their families experiencing these diseases. These modules examine the incidence of each disease process, the pathophysiology of the illness, appropriate assessment techniques and treatments as the disease progresses. The modules further define the psychosocial implications. The modules specifically question the potential ethical, economic and research implications as related to each specific disease process. Each module was written by nursing experts in the field and then reviewed by other expert clinicians of various disciplines to insure you the reader gain the best insight to helping your patients achieve the best the quality of life possible.

Patrick J. Coyne, MSN, APRN, BC-PCM, FAAN
Clinical Director of Thomas Palliative Care Program
Virginia Commonwealth University/Massey Cancer Center
Richmond, VA

James is a 67-year-old man with a 60 pack/year history of cigarette smoking. He tells you he started with unfiltered Camels™ when he was a teenager and switched to filters in the 70s. "Can't quit now . . . I'm too hooked" he tells you as he pauses for breath every two or three words. "I'll probably die . . . with a smoke in my hand . . . he . . . he . . . he" he laughs. "Trouble is . . . I need . . . some relief . . . so I can get . . . around my room."

Overview

Chronic pulmonary diseases are the 4th leading cause of death for all persons who die each year in the United States and pneumonia is the 5th leading cause for persons older than 65 years.[1] The World Health Organization predicts that by 2020 Chronic Obstructive Pulmonary Disease (COPD) will rise from the 12th most prevalent disease worldwide to the 5th and from the 6th most common cause of death to the 3rd.[2] The resulting dyspnea, respiratory distress, cough and secretions burden the patient and are the emphases of palliative care for terminal pulmonary disease.

Chronic pulmonary diseases are those that often have an insidious onset, progress over a period of months to years and can be supported but not cured. Supportive treatments are those that promote respiratory stability and extend the person's life. Similarly, palliative interventions reduce symptom distress and some pulmonary supportive treatments are indistinguishable from palliative interventions, such as oxygen and bronchodilators. COPD is the most common chronic disease referred for terminal symptom management and will be described in this book.

Additionally, pneumonia and aspiration pneumonitis will receive attention as they are the most common acute pulmonary disorders often resulting in the death of patients with chronic or terminal illnesses such as dementia, advanced cancer or neurological conditions.[3] Patients with heart failure and some neurological conditions, such as amyotrophic lateral sclerosis (ALS) or stroke, often succumb from respiratory failure but these disorders will be discussed elsewhere (see *Compendium of End Stage Non-cancer Diagnoses: Neurological Diseases and Trauma*).

While lung replacement technologies such as mechanical ventilation and non-invasive positive pressure ventilation (NIPPV) are commonly used to improve oxygenation and blood gases when the patient has respiratory failure, some patients with terminal disease will forgo these treatments and clinicians are obliged to relieve the symptoms of respiratory failure through other palliative strategies. Rarely, patients may require palliative sedation as an alternative of last resort for refractory respiratory distress.

Mechanical ventilation replaces spontaneous breathing through the delivery of volume, oxygen and humidification using positive pressure. The patient must have an artificial airway such as an oral or nasal endotracheal tube or a tracheostomy. NIPPV is a non-invasive variation of mechanical ventilation that uses positive pressure through a nasal or full face mask when the patient can protect his or her own airway, manage secretions and tolerate the discomfort of the mask.[4] Mechanical ventilation is one of the most burdensome interventions to treat respiratory failure and when the patient is dying from pulmonary disease. The burden of mechanical ventilation is weighed against the patient's values about having life extended through these means.[5] Principles of palliative care should be used when decisions are made to withdraw either form of mechanical ventilation.[6]

> *James is back in the hospital with exacerbation of COPD. He was recently discharged after a two-week hospitalization including five days in the medical ICU requiring intubation and mechanical ventilation. He reported at this hospital admission that he would accept any treatment necessary to reduce his breathlessness, except intubation and ventilation. "I never want that . . . big pipe . . . down my throat . . . again. Anything but that . . . ."*

DEFINITIONS

COPD is characterized by the progressive development of airflow limitation that is not reversible and it encompasses chronic obstructive bronchitis, emphysema and mucus plugging. Most patients with COPD have all three conditions.[7] COPD affects 14 to 20 million Americans each year.[8]

Pneumonia is an infectious process in the lungs, most often bacterial. There are approximately 2.5 million cases per year in the United States. *Aspiration pneumonitis* is a pulmonary chemical injury induced by the aspiration of gastric contents, oropharyngeal secretions or inflammatory exogenous liquids, such as tube feedings.[9,10]

Dyspnea is the most common symptom characterizing pulmonary pathophysiology and is a person's subjective awareness of altered or uncomfortable breathing. *Symptoms* are subjective data that can be perceived and verified by the person experiencing them. The presence and severity of dyspnea is elicited from the patient using a self-report measure.

Respiratory distress has been conceptualized as an observable corollary to dyspnea and defined as the physical and/or emotional suffering that results from the experience of dyspnea. Respiratory distress is characterized by behaviors that can be observed and measured by others even in the absence of a validating report from the patient.[11]

Cough is a natural defense to prevent entry of foreign material into the respiratory tract. It can be a debilitating symptom in patients with chronic or terminal diseases leading to sleeplessness, fatigue, chest pain and sometimes pathological fractures.[12]

Retained upper airway secretions are commonly noted in patients who are near death and have been characterized as a "death rattle." Noisy, moist breathing is produced by an accumulation of salivary and/or bronchial secretions when the patient is too weak to cough effectively. Air passing through the secretions causes the rattling or gurgling sound. Most reports from patients indicate that it is not uncomfortable or distressing.[12]

PATHOPHYSIOLOGY

Chronic Obstructive Pulmonary Disease

Cigarette smoking is the leading cause of COPD in industrialized countries; environmental pollutants are important causes in developing countries. It is likely that there are interactions between environmental factors and a genetic predisposition to COPD, which makes some people more prone to develop COPD than others. There is a chronic inflammatory process in COPD that differs from that seen with asthma.[7,13] Irritants deposited in the lower respiratory tract from cigarette smoke or pollutants and the resulting histopathological responses produce alveolar wall destruction (emphysema) and mucus hypersecretion (chronic bronchitis). Quitting smoking slows but does not appear to halt the inflammatory process in the airways suggesting that there are perpetuating mechanisms once inflammation has become established.[14]

Over time, the person with COPD develops a chronic cough, changes in the volume, tenacity and purulence of sputum and declines in pulmonary function. Many will develop weight loss and fatigue since they cannot eat when they are short of breath. The lungs become hyperinflated, which produces an increased anterior-posterior thoracic diameter (barrel-chest), increased retrosternal airspace, bullae and hilar vascular prominence. Hypoxemia, hypercarbia and reduced peak expiratory flow rate develop.[15]

Advanced stage disease is characterized by a continued decline in respiratory status, decreased ability to complete activities of daily living and frequent emergency department visits or hospital admissions with acute exacerbations. In addition, right sided heart failure and atrial arrhythmias may develop.[16] Reliable prediction of a survival interval of less than six months is not possible with existing tools or guidelines[8,17] as seen in a study that tested the currently available criteria.[18] Even an episode of respiratory failure requiring mechanical ventilation does not by itself predict death within 6 or 12 months.[19] Thus, each acute exacerbation could be the final illness when the patient has severe COPD and decisions about rescue with mechanical ventilation may be determinative in identifying the relevance of a treatment plan in which palliative care interventions are the focus of treatment.

Pneumonia

The most common cause of pneumonia in adults is the aspiration of oropharyngeal secretions or gastric contents, especially in the presence of dysphagia. Risk for aspiration is increased when the patient has depressed consciousness (e.g., stroke, seizure, dementia), neuromuscular disorders that impair swallowing, gastroesophageal reflux or retained upper airway secretions. The development of the infectious process in the lungs after clinical or subclinical aspiration is increased when the patient has impaired immunity, impaired volitional cough, malnutrition and underlying lung disease.

Pneumonia is classified by site of acquisition and host factors. Pneumonia is community-acquired if the onset is within 96 hours of hospital admission and as hospital-acquired (nosocomial) if the onset occurs more than 96 hours after hospital admission. The most typical pathogens are gram-positive cocci (streptococcus pneumonia, Staphylococcus aureus and Enterococcus faecalis), gram-positive bacilli and gram-negative bacilli (H. influenzae, Pseudomonas aeruginosa, E. coli, Proteus mirabilis and Serratia marcescens). Fungi are common in patients who are immunosuppressed.[9,10] The mortality rate of pneumonia remains low in the outpatient setting (1-5%) but climbs to 12% when the patient requires hospitalization and approaches 40% in those who are most ill such as those with bacteremia and from nursing home settings.[20]

Aspiration Pneumonitis

Aspiration pneumonitis is uncommon in healthy individuals and the character and volume of the aspirate predicts the severity of the pulmonary reaction. When there is a large volume of gastric contents aspirated into the airway a cascade of pathophysiological events occur. Initially, there is an epithelial denudation of the trachea with late desquamation followed by inflammatory bronchiolitis. In the alveoli inflammatory exudates form along with microhemorrhages and the production of interstitial edema causing pneumocyte degeneration and hyaline membrane formation. These pathologies contribute to ventilation-perfusion mismatching, intrapulmonary shunting, surfactant loss and atelectasis with pulmonary edema and bronchospasm causing hypoxemia. Superinfection often occurs 2-10 days after aspiration and substantially increases mortality.[10,21]

Cough

Cough is a violent exhalation with flow rates that are high enough to sheer mucus and foreign particles away from the large airways. This reflex to stimulation of the large airways is mediated by the vagus nerve. Bronchial hyperreactivity is indicated by wheezing and cough. Wheezing is produced by irritants, inflammation and excess secretions.[12]

Retained Airway Secretions

The mucociliary transport system inhibits the entrance of viruses, bacteria and other particulate matter into the lower respiratory tract. The surface of the respiratory tract is lined with mucus that is constantly propelled upward toward the oropharynx by ciliated epithelial cells found everywhere in the respiratory tract except the alveoli, nose and throat. The secretions are subconsciously swallowed or coughed out. Excessive accumulation can occur when there is excessive secretion of respiratory mucus, abnormal secretions, dysfunction of the cilia, inability to swallow and decreased cough. Cigarette smoke decreases the activity of the cilia.[12]

ASSESSMENT

Dyspnea and Respiratory Distress

The gold standard for measuring symptom distress is the patient's report. When this is possible in the chronically or terminally ill patient a numeric score similar to that used for pain assessment anchored by "0" for no dyspnea to "100" for the most severe dyspnea may be helpful to trend the patient's response to treatment. While horizontal visual analog scales have been used to assess pain, vertical visual analog scales anchored from 0 to 100 have been useful for measuring dyspnea in cognitively intact patients.[22-24] Concordance with the family's perspective about the patient's behavior and level of comfort should be sought. However, proxy reports about respiratory distress when the patient is unable to provide a self-report may be less reliable than reliance on behavioral cues.[25,26]

Declining or impaired cognition are highly prevalent among terminally ill patients, particularly those who are elderly or referred from long-term care.[3,27] Likewise, hypoxemia will temporarily impair cognition particularly if the PaO_2 is less than 50 mm Hg[28] and hypercarbia produces a narcotic effect at $PaCO_2$ levels >70 mm Hg.[29-31] Patients with COPD who experience chronic blood gas alterations are likely to have mild cognitive impairment even when their oxygenation is stable with declines from baseline occurring when they are hypoxemic.[32-34]

Patients with declining or impaired cognition are vulnerable to under-recognition and under-treatment of their distress because clinicians may lack the ability to identify behavioral responses associated with the autonomic and emotional responses. In fact, investigators recently identified a high frequency of respiratory distress and dyspnea in long-term care. A retrospective audit of 185 charts from five long-term care facilities in

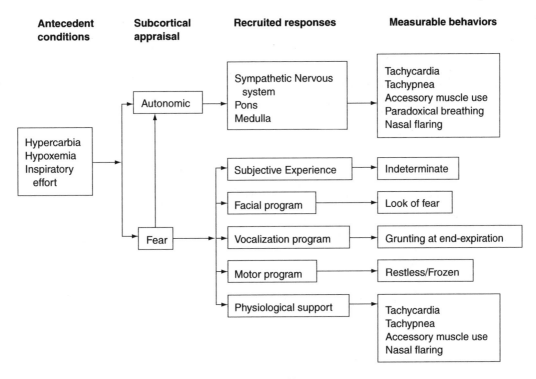

Figure 1   Respiratory Distress Observation Model[26]

Canada found that half of the residents who died were cognitively impaired and dyspnea was the most common symptom (62%) but only 23% of residents with dyspnea had it treated.[27] A corresponding result was found in a large mortality follow back survey of family members of patients who died in an institutional setting. Families reported that 22% of patients with dyspnea did not receive any or enough treatment.[35]

Campbell and Therrien[26] developed a Respiratory Distress Observation Model for the cognitively impaired patient that relies on subcortical neurological systems in the emotional and autonomic domains that are rapidly triggered in response to a threat of asphyxia (see Figure 1). These evolutionary ancient reactions produce compensatory responses oriented to survival.[36] Conditions that produce dyspnea (inspiratory effort, hypercarbia and hypoxemia) trigger a near immediate autonomic and primal emotional reaction (fear) that produces an array of response tendencies that are observable behaviors.

Fear has been strongly correlated with dyspnea in studies of patients with respiratory disease.[26,37-40] The subcortical fear emotion centers are activated in response to a dyspnea antecedent as demonstrated in a number of brain imaging studies.[41-43] Elicitation of fear produces an organized response array of facial (see Figure 2), vocal, motor and physiological responses that can be observed as measurable behaviors. Likewise, the near immediate activation of the autonomic responses from the sympathetic nervous system, adrenal medulla and the ventromedial pons that are both directly activated and triggered by the fear response also produces measurable behaviors.

A recent study of the Respiratory Distress Observation Model identified behavioral correlates of respiratory distress in patients undergoing a weaning trial from mechanical ventilation. The study participants were at risk for weaning failure and displayed a number of signs

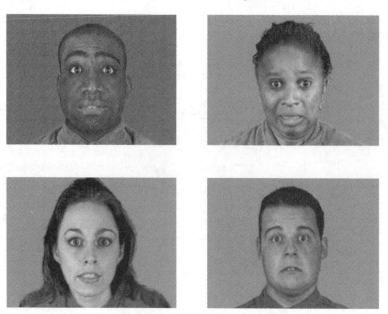

Figure 2   Expressions of primal fear

Used with permission. Beaupre' MG, Cheung N, Hess H. La reconnaisance des expressions emotionelles faciales par des decodeurs africains, asiatiques et caucasiens. Paper presented at: 2nd annual conference of La Societee Quebecoise de recherche en psychologie, 2000.

of respiratory distress, including: tachycardia, tachypnea, accessory muscle use, paradoxical breathing (diaphragmatic), nasal flaring and a fearful facial expression.[26] These behaviors are activated when one or more of hypoxemia, hypercarbia or inspiratory effort triggers pulmonary stress and fear responses. Accessory muscle use is recognized when there is a rise in the clavicles during inspiration. Paradoxical breathing is the outward movement of the abdominal wall during inspiration and is easier to observe when the patient is in bed in a semi-Fowler's position or supine. Thus, assessing dyspnea or respiratory distress when the patient is dying begins with providing the patient with an opportunity to provide a self-report and relying on behavioral cues when a self-report is not possible or is unreliable.

Cough and Retained Airway Secretions

Assessment should be directed at determining the most likely cause, which will guide the choice of treatment. What factors increase cough or secretions, likewise what factors are likely to decrease them? Can the patient clear airway and oropharyngeal secretions? Is the volume or tenacity of the secretions interfering with air flow?

> *James is able to use a vertical dyspnea visual analog scale and he reports his dyspnea ranges from 50-70 on a 0-100 scale. The nurse observes that at 50, James displays accessory muscle use and tachypnea; and he can speak in complete sentences before pausing for breath. When he is more dyspneic, he displays paradoxical breathing in addition to accessory muscle use and tachypnea and he needs to pause for breath after only two or three words. Chest congestion is audible without a stethoscope but clears after James coughs and spits. He reports that he coughs more in the morning and after attempting to lay flat and his cough improves with upright positioning.*

EARLY TREATMENT INTERVENTIONS

Stable COPD

Treatment of stable COPD is largely supportive and palliative and is directed at delaying progression, optimizing lung function and minimizing symptom distress. Smoking cessation is the only measure that will slow the progression of COPD and is aided by nicotine-replacement therapies. None of the existing medications for COPD modify the long-term decline in lung function, thus medications are used to decrease symptoms and/or complications.[44]

Inhaled bronchodilators are the mainstay of current drug therapy for COPD. They are given on an as-needed basis or on a regular basis to prevent or reduce symptoms. The principle bronchodilator treatments are short and long-acting β_2-agonists (albuterol, salmeterol), anticholinergics (ipratropium) and theophylline usually used in combination. While theophylline is effective in treating COPD, inhaled bronchodilators are preferred because of the potential toxicity from theophylline.[44]

Antibiotics are important during acute exacerbations only if a bacterial infection is detected. There is no evidence to support the use of prophylactic antibiotics in COPD.[7] Long-term oxygen therapy (>15 hours/daily) reduced mortality and improved the quality of life in patients with severe COPD who had chronic hypoxemia ($PaO_2 <55$ mm Hg).[45]

Pulmonary rehabilitation is a structured program of education, exercise and physical therapy directed at helping COPD patients master their symptoms, increase exercise capacity and improve quality of life. Lung function does not improve with pulmonary rehabilitation however nurse investigators demonstrated health-related quality-of-life improvements.[46-48]

Lung volume reduction surgery reduces hyperinflation making respiratory muscles more effective. In addition, the elastic recoil of the lung is increased improving expiratory flow. Life expectancy is not improved but exercise capacity and global health status are improved. Lung transplantation for very advanced COPD has been shown to improve quality of life and functional capacity; however this intervention is limited by organ shortages, peri-operative mortality, post-operative complications and the high cost associated with this intervention.[44]

An acute exacerbation of COPD is characterized by some combination of three clinical findings: worsening dyspnea, increase in sputum purulence and increase in sputum volume.[49] Acute exacerbations represent a life-threatening decline often complicated by respiratory failure and sometimes death.[50] The major etiological factors for an acute exacerbation include: viral or bacterial infections, pollution, illness severity and low body mass index.[44,49,50] Acute exacerbations are treated by maximizing the patient's regimen of bronchodilators, anticholinergics and oxygen. A brief course of intravenous corticosteroids followed by oral prednisone tapered over days has been successful in stabilizing patients with acute exacerbations. Mechanical ventilation is indicated when patient fatigue or respiratory failure are present, unless the patient refuses this level of support. NIPPV is less burdensome than intubation and ventilation and is employed if the patient is alert, cooperative, hemodynamically stable, able to maintain his or her own airway and secretions and able to tolerate the mask.[15]

Pneumonia and Pneumonitis

Antibiotic therapy is standard for the treatment of lung infection and may be useful for the patient who is not near death. Supplemental oxygen may be a therapeutic adjunct if the patient is hypoxemic and reporting or displaying respiratory distress.[9] Antibiotics are not routinely given for aspiration pneumonitis unless or until a superinfection develops but bronchodilators and steroids may be therapeutic for treating the associated bronchospasm.[10]

Dyspnea and Respiratory Distress

Treatment of dyspnea or respiratory distress can be organized into three categories: prevention, treatment of the underlying cause and palliation of the symptom distress. Prevention of dyspnea warrants maximizing treatments that have proven beneficial to the patient, including enhancing ventilator synchrony if the patient is going to remain ventilated or use NIPPV, avoiding volume overload and continuing oxygen, nebulized bronchodilators and steroids.

Treating underlying causes of dyspnea may be useful particularly when the benefit of the treatment is not in disproportion to the burden. When death is not imminent the patient may benefit from antibiotics, corticosteroids and bronchoscopy to clear mucus plugs. Draining pleural or pericardial effusions or ascites will also produce dyspnea relief.

Palliation of symptom distress as the major emphasis of care will be discussed in the section **Later Treatment Interventions** that address the care of patients who have severe advanced disease or are near death.

Cough

Cough can lead to sleeplessness, fatigue, disability and sometimes pathological fractures. Treatment of chronic cough will depend on the etiology and the goals of cough treatment may be to reduce the underlying cause verses suppress the symptom. Cough suppressants (opioids and antitussive agents) could be harmful if the COPD patient has excessive secretions and will increase respiratory distress by reducing the patient's ability to expel secretions. Expectorants, humidification and mucolytics will decrease mucus production and improve the patient's ability to clear the airway.[12]

LATER TREATMENT INTERVENTIONS

When the patient with end stage pulmonary disease reaches the active dying phase treatment goals shift from a supportive-prolongative-palliative plan to primarily palliative interventions, although continuation of bronchodilators, steroids and oxygen will reduce symptom distress. Thus, the primary focus shifts from treating the disease process to treating the distressing symptoms.

Terminal Dyspnea and Respiratory Distress

A number of strategies have demonstrated effectiveness for palliation of terminal dyspnea including optimal positioning, oxygen and sitting in front of a fan. Upright positioning with arms elevated and supported affords the patient an optimal lung capacity and is useful when caring for a patient with COPD.[51,52] Oxygen has been shown to be more effective than air in patients with an advanced stage COPD[53] and increased ambient air flow, fans and cold air have also been therapeutic.[54-57] Oxygen can be more burdensome than beneficial in the patient who is near death, particularly when face masks are employed since the mask produces a feeling of suffocation. Reliance on the patient's report or behavior in response to oxygen will guide decisions about its usefulness. High dose oxygen can contribute to hypoventilation and worsening hypercarbia in the COPD patient,[58] however, hypercarbia does not increase distress particularly when CO_2 levels exceed 70 mm Hg.

Opioids, most commonly morphine or fentanyl, are the mainstay of pharmacological management of terminal dyspnea and effectiveness has been demonstrated in numerous clinical trials. A meta-analysis of eighteen studies that were double blind, randomized, placebo controlled trials of opioids in the treatment of dyspnea from any cause revealed a statistically positive effect on the sensation of breathlessness (p=0.0008). Meta-regression indicated a greater effect for studies using oral or parenteral opioids than for studies using nebulized opioids with approximately the same results found when COPD studies were compared to cancer studies.[59] Doses for treating dyspnea are patient-specific, generally lower than those needed to relieve pain and as with opioid use in managing pain; no ceiling should be placed on dosage. Close bedside evaluation to assess the efficacy of the medication is essential.

Fear and anxiety may be components of the respiratory distress experienced by the dying patient. The addition of a benzodiazepine to the opioid regimen has been successful in patients with advanced COPD.[60] As with opioids, these agents should be titrated to effect.

Patients may choose to have their life extended with mechanical ventilation and/or NIPPV. Likewise, after a trial of these interventions the patient may make a decision to have ventilation withdrawn.

Cough and Retained Airway Secretions

Opioids and/or inhaled anesthetic lidocaine are indicated to suppress non-productive cough when the patient is actively dying. Retained airway secretions can be managed by changing the patient's position to promote drainage, reducing or eliminating intravenous hydration and topical, subcutaneous or parenteral anticholinergic drugs such as glycopyrrolate and scopolamine. Suctioning is not recommended unless there is a large volume of easily reached secretions since it is such a burdensome intervention.[12]

> *James has been admitted with an acute exacerbation of COPD and has affirmed his refusal of intubation and mechanical ventilation. On a 0-100 dyspnea visual analog scale (DVAS) he reports his dyspnea severity at 90 and he is displaying accessory muscle use, tachypnea, tachycardia, paradoxical breathing and a fearful facial expression. Very poor air exchange is noted on chest auscultation. His arterial blood gases reveal pH 7.10, PO_2 42, PCO_2 80, Bicarbonate 38 and SO_2 of 79% on a 100% non-rebreather mask.*
>
> *He is receiving aerosolized albuterol and ipratropium every four hours, methylPREDNISolone intravenously every six hours and oxygen. He agrees to a trial of NIPPV but finds the face mask to be so unpleasant that after six hours he asks for it to be removed.*
>
> *He knows he may be dying and agrees to whatever strategies may be helpful to reduce his severe respiratory distress. He continues to refuse intubation. A "DNR-comfort measures only" order is entered in his record. Bronchodilators and steroids are continued. Additionally, James receives 1 mg of lorazepam and 3 mg of morphine given as intravenous boluses. After 5 minutes, James reports that his DVAS is 70 and while he continues to display accessory muscle use and tachypnea, he is less tachycardic and is no longer showing paradoxical breathing or facial fear. His oxygen saturation has risen from 79% to 90% and he tolerates a change from a 100% non-rebreather to nasal cannula at 2 l/min.*

Over the next 48 hours James reports a DVAS average at 50 and maintains his oxygen saturation between 88 and 92% on nasal cannula. He receives lorazepam 1 mg every six hours around-the-clock and rapid release oral morphine 10 mg every 1 hour as needed for breakthrough dyspnea. He needs the morphine when he is active, such as while bathing or when getting up to the bathroom.

On the fourth hospital day, James leaves the hospital to go to his sister's home and he has accepted a referral for hospice care.

Ventilator Withdrawal

Ventilator withdrawal is a process of liberating a terminally ill patient from mechanical ventilation recognizing that patient death may follow in minutes to days. Preventing or reducing respiratory distress before, during and after ventilator withdrawal is a priority. The patient's ability to experience distress predicts the most optimal method for withdrawal. Ventilator withdrawal is comprised of three processes: pre-medication, withdrawal method and extubation. Decisions are made about each of these processes that allow the withdrawal to be individually tailored to the patient's unique clinical circumstances and personal requirements. A single method is not sufficiently patient-centered.

ADVANCE PREPARATIONS

Prior to beginning the withdrawal process, the clinician has an opportunity to create a therapeutic milieu and to meet patient or family needs for counseling, religious or cultural rituals or other life-closure tasks. Awake patients should have the withdrawal process explained and should know what sensations to expect. Likewise, the patient must know that the team will direct all their activities during withdrawal to ensuring respiratory comfort. Families will have similar needs for information.[61]

Additionally, some mechanically ventilated ICU patients are paralyzed with neuromuscular blocking agents (NMBA) to achieve patient-ventilator synchrony and to minimize tissue oxygen consumption. Discontinuation of NMBA before ventilator withdrawal is essential since the paralyzed patient will not be able to display signs of distress until the medication wears off; clinicians will have no patient report or behavioral cues to guide assessment of respiratory comfort. Likewise, the patient might be awake and will experience apnea if they remain paralyzed for the withdrawal process.[62-64]

PRE-MEDICATION

Patients may be pre-medicated before ventilator withdrawal when respiratory distress can be anticipated since pre-medication will prevent development of distress. Pre-medication agents include morphine for its known properties for treating dyspnea and a sedating agent such as a benzodiazepine or barbiturate may be given as an adjunct. All patients will not require pre-medication before ventilator withdrawal. The patient who is awake will be able to negotiate sedation goals with the clinician taking into consideration the patient's likelihood of experiencing respiratory distress. For example, a patient who is alert but has a C-2 quadriplegia with no ability for spontaneous ventilation after ventilator withdrawal is going to need complete anesthesia while a COPD patient with marginal pulmonary parameters may need little sedation initially.

Many patients undergoing ventilator withdrawal are unconscious from direct neurological insults or from the consequences of organ failure; comatose and brain dead patients do not require pre-medication.[65,66] Thus, pre-medication should be considered for patients with signs of respiratory distress before ventilator withdrawal and patients at-risk for respiratory distress during or after ventilator withdrawal.

Standardized doses of opioids and benzodiazepines have not been established for dyspnea treatment in this context. A suggested dose for pre-medication with morphine is a bolus of 5-10 mg if the patient is opioid naïve, however, illness severity and tolerance will influence dosing. Respiratory comfort is maintained with a continuous infusion at a rate equal to 50% of the bolus dose. Lorazepam (2-4 mg) or midazolam (2-5 mg) are useful adjuncts if anxiolysis or amnesia is desired.[67] Propofol or a barbiturate is useful if palliative sedation is indicated.[68,69] Treatment with scopolamine or glycopyrrolate intravenously prior to ventilator withdrawal may reduce excessive secretions that could pose a burden if the patient is extubated.

WITHDRAWAL METHOD
Terminal weaning entails a reduction in oxygen and ventilatory support incrementally over a period of 15-20 minutes. This method affords the most control and should be employed when the patient is at-risk for respiratory distress. The process can be stopped at any time during weaning to adjust the patient's medications if signs of distress appear. This method is indicated whenever a patient is at-risk for respiratory distress during or after ventilator withdrawal.

The following steps comprise terminal weaning

1. Pre-medicate, if indicated, then begin a continuous infusion of the pre-medicant;
2. Decrease PEEP, FiO$_2$ and minute volume of ventilation incrementally over 15-20 minutes. Observe the patient continuously for signs of distress;
3. Stop the process to re-bolus and titrate medication if signs of distress are apparent;
4. Conclude the wean with placing the patient on a t-piece with humidified room air or oxygen.

Immediate t-piece placement is a satisfactory withdrawal method when the patient is unlikely to experience respiratory distress because of severely impaired cognition or coma. The following steps comprise immediate t-piece placement

1. Pre-medicate, if indicated;
2. Turn off ventilator and place patient on a t-piece with humidified room air;
3. Medicate the patient if signs of distress develop after ventilator withdrawal.

EXTUBATION
Patients who will experience distress from a nasal or oral endotracheal tube should be extubated. Patient's may need to retain their tube if there is a large volume of pulmonary secretions, impaired or absent gag/cough reflexes, a swollen or protuberant tongue, inhalation injury or high risk for post-extubation stridor. Balancing burden with benefit will determine when the patient should be extubated. Post-extubation stridor or laryngospasm can be reduced with the application of an aerosol mask and administration of nebulized racemic epinephrine. Table 1 provides withdrawal suggestions for common clinical circumstances.

Although this book focuses on COPD, other debilitating illnesses may produce respiratory failure as the terminal condition. Thus, case examples of patients with ALS and stroke are provided. Detailed care of patients with neurological illnesses is published elsewhere (see Compendium of End Stage Non-cancer Diagnoses: Neurological Diseases and Trauma).

TABLE 1   Processes for Withdrawal of Mechanical Ventilation Under Various Clinical Circumstances

Clinical Condition	Pre-medication	Withdrawal Method	Extubation	Oxygen after Withdrawal	Clinical Rationale
C1-C4 quadriplegia	Propofol or barbituate to achieve deep anesthesia	Immediated t-bar with room air	Yes	No	Patient will be apneic, complete sedation is essential
COPD & awake	Negotiate goals with patient. Morphine or morphine & benzodiazepine	Rapid weaning	Yes	Yes, if awake & reports/displays comfort from oxygen	
ARDS	Discontinue NMBA. Evaluate ability to experience distress after NMBA wears off. Morphine & benzodiazepine	Rapid weaning. Wean PEEP & FiO_2 first	Evaluate risk for post-extubation stridor. Evaluate volume of pulmonary secretions	Yes, if awake & able to experience comfort from oxygen	Poor pulmonary compliance will make spontaneous breaths labored, thus ventilation is weaned last
Pneumonia & dementia	Morphine & benzodiazepine	Rapid weaning	Yes	Yes, if signs of respiratory distress are reduced with nasal oxygen	
Comatose	None	Immediate t-piece	No, unless gag & cough reflexes are intact	No	Patient cannot experience distress. Disconcerting airway sounds may occur if patient is extubated
Brain dead	None	Immediate t-piece	Yes	No	Patient is dead & cannot experience distress & will not display airway difficulties

ARDS – Adult Respiratory Distress Syndrome, PEEP – positive end-expiratory pressure, NMBA – neuromuscular blocking agent, FiO_2 – fraction of inspired oxygen

CASE EXAMPLE: VENTILATOR WITHDRAWAL AND ALS

Carol is admitted via the Emergency Department to the MICU in acute respiratory failure. She was intubated en route to the hospital by the paramedics. Carol is in the terminal stage of amyotrophic lateral sclerosis (ALS) and had been referred by her neurologist for hospice care but the initial hospice visit had not occurred when Carol became severely dyspneic and her husband called 911.

After stabilization in the MICU, Carol communicated her wishes to have ventilation withdrawn. Her husband and neurologist validated that Carol had previously decided to forgo ventilation when her ALS reached the respiratory failure stage. Carol and her family were counseled that her survival duration off the ventilator might be measured in minutes to hours and that Carol's respiratory comfort would be the priority of care. The ventilator withdrawal was postponed for 24 hours to afford Carol and her husband, children and other family members unrestricted opportunities for life closure activities. The hospital chaplain worked closely with Carol and her family during this interval.

Carol's pulmonary parameters were very poor and suggestive of a high probability of respiratory distress when ventilation was reduced. Carol indicated her preference to be "asleep"; she feared another episode of breathlessness. After spending a quiet interval alone with her husband, a continuous propofol infusion was started and within minutes Carol was unresponsive.

Terminal weaning was initiated and over 15 minutes the FiO_2 was weaned to room air and ventilation was weaned until Carol was breathing spontaneously through the ventilator. The nurse and respiratory therapist remained at the bedside during weaning to closely monitor Carol for signs of re-awakening and respiratory distress and to support her family who had remained at the bedside.

The ventilator was turned off and Carol's oral endotracheal tube was removed. She breathed spontaneously and her respirations were rapid and very shallow as expected.

Carol's oxygen saturation dropped but there were no signs of re-awakening or respiratory distress. She died 20 minutes after the ventilator was discontinued.

CASE EXAMPLE: VENTILATOR WITHDRAWAL AND STROKE

Leonard was found unresponsive in his apartment by his landlord. Admission to the hospital and work-up disclosed an acute hemorrhagic stroke with mass effect producing coma. A poor prognosis for functional neurologic recovery was predicted by the neurointensivist in consultation with a neurosurgeon.

Leonard's family agreed with the physician's recommendation to change treatment goals to comfort care and to withdraw mechanical ventilation.

Leonard was comatose with no brainstem reflexes except a weak cough. His family was counseled that duration of survival after ventilator withdrawal could not be

(continued)

reliably predicted but would probably occur in 24 to 48 hours after the ventilator was discontinued. His family said their "good-byes" to Leonard and chose to leave the hospital and remain in contact by telephone.

Leonard required no pre-medication and his ventilator was withdrawn by immediate t-piece placement. His tongue was swollen, gag reflex was absent and cough reflex was weak so the oral endotracheal tube was left in place to t-piece with humidified room air. Leonard displayed no signs of respiratory distress and his respiratory pattern was consistent with Cheyne-Stokes breathing. He died 32 hours after the ventilator was withdrawn.

PSYCHOSOCIAL

COPD patients have a high prevalence of generalized anxiety disorder, depression and panic attacks compared to the general population.[40] Prior to the terminal stage antidepressant therapy, particularly the SSRIs, alleviate anxiety and reduce panic disorder.[70] However, therapeutic effects are not often seen until two to four weeks after treatment initiation, thus benzodiazepines may be the most useful agent to reduce the psychological symptoms associated with acute dyspnea. Likewise, even when treatment with an antidepressant is adequate, benzodiazepines may still be necessary particularly during acute exacerbations. As with opioids, these agents should be titrated to effect. Acute withdrawal of benzodiazepines may occur when the patient experiences difficulty swallowing or is actively dying and withdrawal symptoms (anxiety, nausea, agitation) may develop. Care should be taken to ensure the maintenance of these agents by employing alternative routes of administration (subcutaneous or intravenous) when oral administration is not possible.

As COPD progresses the increasing pulmonary disability leads to a number of detrimental effects. Frustration and fatigue were identified as common shared experiences of patient's living with COPD. Functional disabilities produce difficulty in previously 'taken for granted' activities of daily living, such as bathing, bending to tie shoelaces and leaving the house. Patients are concerned about their image if they must use a wheelchair or wear oxygen in public causing some to stay home, which leads to social isolation. Patients reported that being housebound led to losses such as loss of occupation from early retirement, loss of family and other social relationships and loss of intimacy. Guilt from smoking was not identified, but patients acknowledged that their disease was 'self-inflicted' but justified smoking because "we were not aware of the health damage it could do."[71] Some patients with advanced pulmonary disease are unable or unwilling to quit smoking in spite of counseling and must be taught how to smoke safely when they are using long-term oxygen.

Coping interventions for the detrimental effects of COPD focus on activity modification and energy conservation, social support and support groups. Patients are taught, often in pulmonary rehabilitation programs, how to modify tasks to reduce breathlessness by pacing their activities or by substituting pleasurable hobbies that produce less effort, such as cards instead of golf. Resting before eating, substituting small, frequent meals for large meals and sipping liquid supplements reduces energy expenditure during meals. Social support must be timed and matched to the person's needs. For instance, some patients isolate themselves because their dyspnea prevents them from participating in social activities.[72]

Family caregivers assume increased burden as the patient's disability increases. A qualitative study of wives caring for husbands with COPD revealed a number of positive and negative themes. Negative aspects included: physical fatigue, interrupted sleep due to nighttime vigilance regarding husband's condition, weakening of marital intimacy, depression and feelings of isolation. Positive factors were having employment outside the home, spiritual strength and duty to care for their husbands "until the end."[73] Support for caregivers can come from referral to home care agencies and to hospice when the patient reaches the terminal stage.

ECONOMICS

COPD is highly prevalent and as it progresses patients become too disabled to work. Thus, there is a substantial economic and social burden associated with COPD. Data from the United States have estimated the total amount of economic burden from COPD at $23.9 billion of which $15 million is for direct medical expenditures and the remaining billions related to morbidity, loss of work and premature death. Unacknowledged and un-quantified costs include the economic value of the care provided by family members and their potential lost wages as they stay home to care for the patient.[74]

As COPD progresses, some patients will choose mechanical ventilation as a prolongative/palliative treatment option. Although the patient with advanced disease is eligible for hospice care, many hospices cannot afford to accept the patient with mechanical ventilation into their program because this high-tech intervention drives the cost of care beyond the standard insurance reimbursement. Thus, patients and families may be deprived of the benefits of hospice care.

ETHICS

Fear of prescribing and administering opioids and/or benzodiazepines in terminal dyspnea occurs because clinicians recognize the possibility of respiratory depression as an adverse effect and want to avoid hastening patient death. Studies about patients' experiences after ventilator withdrawal found no evidence that patient death was hastened by the administration of opioids and sedatives.[66,75,76] Results of these studies suggest that prudent administration of opioids and sedatives titrated to patient effect beginning with low doses does not hasten death. Withholding opioids and sedatives in the face of unrelieved respiratory distress is a moral breach because patients have the right to relief of their suffering.[77-79]

Palliative sedation, also known as complete, total or terminal sedation, is an alternative of last resort for the palliation of any symptom that is refractory to standard treatment and is morally appropriate when all other reasonable approaches to relieve symptom distress have been exhausted.[80] When palliative sedation is employed, the sedating agent is titrated against apparent unconsciousness of the patient. Some argue that palliative sedation is not distinguishable from euthanasia with employment of the principle of double effect in counterargument.[81] While endorsed by the National Hospice and Palliative Care Organization[82] and the Hospice and Palliative Nurses Association[83] this intervention remains controversial.

RESEARCH QUESTIONS

Dyspnea and respiratory distress have not received as much attention as pain in palliative care research and chronic respiratory disorders are not as well studied as lung cancer. Thus, a number of questions about terminal pulmonary disease and its consequences need to be addressed. For example, does the experience of dyspnea vary by underlying patho-physiology? What is the most valid and reliable measure of respiratory distress when the patient can provide a self-report? What is the most valid and reliable measure of respira-tory distress when the patient is cognitively impaired? What is the prevalence of dyspnea and/or respiratory distress in patients who are cognitively impaired at the end of life? What strategies are most useful for treating respiratory distress? How does the treatment vary by diagnosis, stage of illness progression and subject cognition?

SUMMARY

Acute and chronic respiratory diseases are common among patients referred for end-of-life care. Dyspnea, respiratory distress, cough and retained airway secretions burden the patient and are the emphases of a respiratory palliative care treatment plan. Assessment depends on the cognitively intact patient's ability to give a self report and on behavioral cues from the cognitively impaired or comatose patient. Treatments vary by the individ-ual patient goals and the stage of illness progression and may include prolongative thera-pies such as mechanical ventilation. As death becomes imminent, the focus of care is on reducing dyspnea and respiratory distress using non-pharmacologic strategies along with opioids and sedatives. Clinicians are guided in their treatment by available research, prac-tice guidelines and ethical standards.

CITED REFERENCES

1. Center for Disease Control. National Center for Health Statistics. Hyattsville, MD; 2003.

2. Lopez AD, Murray CC. The global burden of disease, 1990-2020. *Nature Medicine.* 1998;4:1241-1243.

3. Brandt HE, Deliens L, Ooms ME, van der Steen JT, van der Wal G, Ribbe MW. Symptoms, signs, problems, and diseases of terminally ill nursing home patients. *Archives of Internal Medicine.* 2005;165:314-320.

4. Chesnutt MS, Papadakos PJ. Respiratory failure. In: Kruse JA, Fink MP, Carlson RW, eds. *Saunders Manual of Critical Care.* Philadelphia, PA: Saunders; 2003:17-19.

5. Campbell ML, Bizek KS. Use of NIPPV in terminal respiratory insufficiency. *American Journal of Critical Care.* 1994;3:250-251.

6. Rubenfeld GD. Principles and practice or withdrawing life-sustaining treatments. *Critical Care Clinics.* 2004;20(3):435-452.

7. Barnes PJ. Chronic obstructive pulmonary disease. *New England Journal of Medicine.* 2000;343:269-280.

8. American Thoracic Society. Standards for the diagnosis and care of patients with chronic obstructive pulmonary disease. *American Journal of Respiratory and Critical Care Medicine.* 1995;152:S77-S121.

9. Szalados JE. Pneumonia in adults. In: Kruse JA, Fink MP, Carlson RW, eds. *Saunders Manual of Critical Care.* Philadelphia, PA: Saunders; 2003:37-41.

10. Szalados JE. Aspiration pneumonitis and pneumonia. In: Kruse JA, Fink MP, Carlson RW, eds. *Saunders Manual of Critical Care.* Philadelphia, PA: Saunders; 2003:42-45.

11. Campbell ML. Terminal dyspnea and respiratory distress. *Critical Care Clinics.* 2004;20(3):403-417.

12. Dudgeon D. Dyspnea, death rattle, and cough. In: Ferrell BR, Coyle N, eds. *Oxford Textbook of Palliative Nursing.* 2nd ed. New York, NY: Oxford University Press; 2006:249-264.

13. Barnes PJ. Mechanisms in COPD: differences from asthma. *CHEST.* 2000;117:10S-14S.

14. Rutgers SR, Postma DS, ten Hacken NHT, et al. Ongoing airway inflammation in patients with COPD who do not currently smoke. *Thorax.* 2000;55:12-18.

15. Apostolakos MJ. COPD exacerbation. In: Kruse JA, Fink MP, Carlson RW, eds. *Saunders Manual of Critical Care.* Philadelphia, PA: Saunders; 2003:46-47.

16. Hansen-Flaschen J. Chronic obstructive pulmonary disease: The last year of life. *Respiratory Care.* 2004;49:90-98.

17. National Hospice Organization. Medical guidelines for determining prognosis in selected non-cancer diseases. *Hospice Journal.* 1996;11:47-63.

18. Fox E, Landrum-McNiff K, Zhong Z, Dawson NV, Wu AW, Lynn J. Evaluation of prognostic criteria for determining hospice eligibility in patients with advanced lung, heart, or liver disease. *JAMA.* 1999;282:1638-1645.

19. Seneff MG, Wagner DP, Wagner RP, Zimmerman JE, Knaus WA. Hospital and 1-year survival of patients admitted to intensive care units with chronic obstructive pulmonary disease. *JAMA.* 1995;274:1852-1857.

20. American Thoracic Society. Guidelines for the management of adults with community-acquired pneumonia. *American Journal of Respiratory and Critical Care Medicine.* 2001;163:1730-1754.

21. Marik PE. Aspiration pneumonitis and pneumonia. *New England Journal of Medicine.* 2001;344:665-671.

22. Gift AG. Clinical measurement of dyspnea. *Dimensions of Critical Care Nursing.* 1989;8(4):210-216.

23. Gift AG, Narsavage G. Validity of the numeric rating scale as a measure of dyspnea. *American Journal of Critical Care.* 1998;7:200-204.

24. Gift A. Validation of a vertical visual analogue scale as a measure of clinical dyspnea. *Rehabilitation Nursing.* 1989;14:323-325.

25. Radbruch L, Sabatowski R, Loick G, et al. Cognitive impairment and its influence on pain and symptom assessment in a palliative care unit: development of a Minimal Documentation System. *Palliative Medicine.* 2000;14:266-276.

26. Campbell ML, Therrien B. Behavioral correlates of respiratory distress activated by subcortical brain areas. Paper presented at: Midwest Nursing Research Society Annual Meeting; April 3, 2005; Cincinnati, OH.

27. Hall P, Schroder C, Weaver L. The last 48 hours of life in long-term care: a focused chart audit. *Journal of the American Geriatric Society.* 2002;50:501-506.

28. Moosavi SH, Golestanian E, Binks AP, Lansing RW, Brown R, Banzett RB. Hypoxic and hypercapnic drives to breathe generate equivalent levels of air hunger in humans. *Journal of Applied Physiology.* 2003;94:141-154.

29. Dean JB, Mulkey DK, Garcia AJ, Putnam RW, Henderson RA. Neuronal sensitivity to hyperoxia, hypercapnia, and inert gases at hyperbaric pressures. *Journal of Applied Physiology.* 2003;95:883-909.

30. Reid KH, Patenaude B, Guo SZ, Iyer VG. Carbon dioxide narcosis-induced apnea in a rat model of cardiac arrest and resuscitation. *Resuscitation.* 1998;38:185-191.

31. Taxen DV. Permissive hypercapnia. In: Tobin MJ, ed. *Principles and Practices of Mechanical Ventilation.* New York, NY: McGraw-Hill Book Co.; 1994.

32. Kozora E, Filley CM, Julian LJ, Cullum CM. Cognitive functioning in patients with chronic obstructive pulmonary disease and mild hypoxemia compared with patients with mild Alzheimer disease and normal controls. *Neuropsychiatry, Neuropsychology, and Behavioral Neurology.* 1999;12(3):178-183.

33. Incalzi RA, Marra C, Giordano A, et al. Cognitive impairment in chronic obstructive pulmonary disease: a neuropsychological and spect study. *Journal of Neurology.* 2003;250:325-332.

34. Liesker JJW, Postma DS, Beukema RJ, et al. Cognitive performance in patients with COPD. *Respiratory Medicine.* 2004;98:351-356.

35. Teno JM, Clarridge BR, Casey V, et al. Family perspectives on end-of-life care at the last place of care. *JAMA.* 2004;291:88-93.

36. Gooden BA. The evolution of asphyxial defense. *Integrative Physiological and Behavioral Science.* 1993;28:317-330.

37. DeVito AJ. Dyspnea during hospitalization for acute phase of illness as recalled by patients with chronic obstructive pulmonary disease. *Heart & Lung.* 1990;19:186-191.

38. Gift AG, Cahill CA. Psychophysiologic aspects of dyspnea in chronic obstructive pulmonary disease: a pilot study. *Heart & Lung.* 1990;19(3):252-257.

39. Kellner R, Samet J, Pathak D. Dyspnea, anxiety, and depression in chronic respiratory impairment. *General Hospital Psychiatry.* 1992;14:20-28.

40. Brenes GA. Anxiety and chronic obstructive pulmonary disease: prevalence, impact, and treatment. *Psychosomatic Medicine.* 2003;65:963-970.

41. Banzett RB, Mulnier HE, Murphy K, Rosen SD, Wise RJ, Adams L. Breathlessness in humans activates insular cortex. *Neuroreport.* 2000;11(10):2117-2120.

42. Brannan S, Liotti M, Egan G, et al. Neuroimaging of cerebral activations and deactivations associated with hypercapnia and hunger for air. *Proceedings of the National Academy of Science.* 2001;98(4):2029-2034.

43. Evans KC, Banzett RB, Adams L, McKay L, Frackowiak RSJ, Corfield DR. BOLD fMRI identifies limbic, paralimbic, and cerebellar activation during air hunger. *Journal of Neurophysiology.* 2002;88:1500-1511.

44. GOLD Expert Panel. Global Initiative for Chronic Obstructive Lung Disease. Available at: *www.goldcopd.org.* Accessed November 3, 2005.

45. Tarpy SP, Celli BR. Long-term oxygen therapy. *New England Journal of Medicine.* 1995;333:710-714.

46. Carrieri-Kohlman V, Gormley JM, Eiser S, et al. Dyspnea and the affective response during exercise training in obstructive pulmonary disease. *Nursing Research.* 2001;50(3):136-146.

47. Hernandez MT, Rubio TM, Ruiz FO, Riera HS, Gil RS, Gomez JC. Results of a home-based training program for patients with COPD. *Chest.* 2000;118(1):106-114.

48. Oh EG. The effects of home-based pulmonary rehabilitation in patients with chronic lung disease. *International Journal of Nursing Studies.* 2003;40:873-879.

49. Snow V, Lascher S, Mottur-Pilson C. Evidence base for management of acute exacerbations of chronic obstructive lung disease. *Annals of Internal Medicine.* 2001;134:595-599.

50. Wouters EFM. Management of severe COPD. *The Lancet.* 2004;364:883-895.

51. Barach AL. Chronic obstructive lung disease: postural relief of dyspnea. *Archives of Physical Medicine and Rehabilitation.* 1974;55:494-504.

52. Sharp JT, Drutz WS, Moisan T, Foster J, Machnach W. Postural relief of dyspnea in severe chronic obstructive lung disease. *American Review of Respiratory Disease.* 1980;122:201-211.

53. Swinburn CR, Mould H, Stone TN, Corris PA, Gibson GJ. Symptomatic benefit of supplemental oxygen in hypoxemic patients with chronic lung disease. *American Review of Respiratory Disease.* 1991;143:913-915.

54. Burgess KR, Whitelaw WA. Reducing ventilatory response to carbon dioxide by breathing cold air. *American Review of Respiratory Disease.* 1984;129:687-690.

55. Burgess KR, Whitelaw WA. Effects of nasal cold receptors on pattern of breathing. *Journal of Applied Physiology.* 1988;64:371-376.

56. Liss HP, Grant BJB. The effect of nasal flow on breathlessness in patients with chronic obstructive pulmonary disease. *American Review of Respiratory Disease.* 1988;137:1285-1288.

57. Schwartzstein RM, Lahive K, Pope A, Weinberger SE, Weiss JW. Cold facial stimulation reduces breathlessness induced in normal subjects. *American Review of Respiratory Disease.* 1987;136:58-61.

58. Wilson RH, Hoseth W, Dempsey ME. Respiratory acidosis: effects of decreasing respiratory minute volume in patients with severe chronic pulmonary emphysema, with specific reference to oxygen, morphine and barbiturates. *American Journal of Medicine.* 1954;October:464-470.

59. Jennings AL, Davies AN, Higgins JP, Gibbs JS, Broadley KE. A systematic review of the use of opioids in the management of dyspnea. *Thorax.* 2002;57:922-923.

60. Light RW, Stansbury DW, Webster JS. Effect of 30mg of morphine alone or with promethazine or prochlorperazine on the exercise capacity of patients with COPD. *Chest.* 1996;109:975-981.

61. Kirchhoff KT, Conradt KL, Anumandia PR. ICU nurses' preparation of families for death of patients following withdrawal of life support. *Applied Nursing Research.* 2003;16:85-92.

62. Truog RD, Burns JP. To breathe or not to breathe. *Journal of Clinical Ethics.* 1994;5(1):39-42.

63. Rushton C, Terry PB. Neuromuscular blockade and ventilator withdrawal: ethical controversies. *American Journal of Critical Care.* 1995;4:112-115.

64. Brody H, Campbell ML, Faber-Langendoen K, Ogle KS. Withdrawing intensive life-sustaining treatment: recommendations for compassionate clinical management. *The New England Journal of Medicine.* 1997;336:652-657.

65. Campbell ML, Thill MC. Impact of patient consciousness on the intensity of the do-not-resuscitate therapeutic plan. *American Journal of Critical Care.* 1996;5:339-345.

66. Campbell ML, Bizek KS, Thill MC. Patient responses during rapid terminal weaning from mechanical ventilation: a prospective study. *Critical Care Medicine.* 1999;27:73-77.

67. Campbell ML. *Forgoing mechanical ventilation. Forgoing life-sustaining therapy: How to care for the patient who is near death.* Aliso Viejo, CA: American Association of Critical-Care Nurses; 1998.

68. Truog RD, Cist AFM, Brackett SE, et al. Recommendations for end-of-life care in the intensive care unit: the ethics committee of the Society of Critical Care Medicine. *Critical Care Medicine.* 2001;29:2332-2348.

69. Jacobi J, Fraser GL, Coursin DB, et al. Clinical practice guidelines for the sustained use of sedatives and analgesics in the critically ill adult. *Critical Care Medicine.* 2002;30:119-141.

70. Periyakoil VS, Skultety K, Sheikh J. Panic, anxiety, and chronic dyspnea. *Journal of Palliative Medicine.* 2005;8:453-459.

71. Barnett M. Chronic obstructive pulmonary disease: a phenomenological study of patients' experiences. *Journal of Clinical Nursing.* 2005;14:805-812.

72. Carrieri-Kohlman V, Gormley JM. Coping strategies for dyspnea. In: Mahler DA, ed. *Dyspnea.* New York, NY: Marcel Dekker, Inc.; 1998:287-320.

73. Bergs D. "The hidden client" - women caring for husbands with COPD: their experience of quality of life. *Journal of Clinical Nursing.* 2002;11:613-621.

74. Daly BJ, Thomas D, Dyer MA. Procedures used in withdrawal of mechanical ventilation. *American Journal of Critical Care.* 1995;5:331-338.

75. Pauwels RA, Rabe KF. Burden and clinical features of chronic obstructive pulmonary disease. *The Lancet.* 2004;364:613-620.

76. Wilson WC, Smedira NG, Fink C, McDowell JA, Luce JM. Ordering and administration of sedatives and analgesics during the withholding and withdrawal of life support from critically ill patients. *Journal of the American Medical Association.* 1992;267:949-953.

77. Beauchamp TL, Childress JF. *Principles of biomedical ethics.* 4th ed. New York, NY: Oxford University Press; 1994.

78. President's Commission for the Study of Ethical Problems in Medicine and Behavioral Research. *Deciding to Forego Life-Sustaining Treatment.* Washington, D.C.: U.S. Government Printing Office; 1983.

79. The Hastings Center. *Guidelines on the Termination of Life-Sustaining Treatment and the Care of the Dying.* Bloomington, IN: Indiana University Press; 1987.

80. Fine P. Total sedation in end-of-life care: clinical considerations. *Journal of Hospice and Palliative Nursing.* 2001;3(3):81-87.

81. Burt RA. The Supreme Court speaks-not assisted suicide but a constitutional right to palliative care. *New England Journal of Medicine.* 1997;337:1234-1236.

82. Committee on Ethics of the National Hospice and Palliative Care Organization. *Total Sedation Educational Resources.* Alexandria, VA: National Hospice and Palliative Care Organization; 2001.

83. Dahlin C, Lynch M. HPNA position statement: Palliative sedation at end of life. *Journal of Hospice and Palliative Nursing.* 2003;5:235-238.